T0237668

Cambridge Elements ☰

Elements of Improving Quality and Safety in Healthcare
edited by
Mary Dixon-Woods,* Katrina Brown,* Sonja Marjanovic,†
Tom Ling,† Ellen Perry,* and Graham Martin*
*THIS Institute (The Healthcare Improvement Studies Institute)
†RAND Europe

GOVERNANCE
AND LEADERSHIP

Naomi J. Fulop and Angus I. G. Ramsay
*Department of Applied Health Research,
University College London*

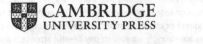

CAMBRIDGE
UNIVERSITY PRESS

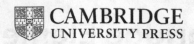

Shaftesbury Road, Cambridge CB2 8EA, United Kingdom

One Liberty Plaza, 20th Floor, New York, NY 10006, USA

477 Williamstown Road, Port Melbourne, VIC 3207, Australia

314–321, 3rd Floor, Plot 3, Splendor Forum, Jasola District Centre,
New Delhi – 110025, India

103 Penang Road, #05–06/07, Visioncrest Commercial, Singapore 238467

Cambridge University Press is part of Cambridge University Press & Assessment,
a department of the University of Cambridge.

We share the University's mission to contribute to society through the pursuit of
education, learning and research at the highest international levels of excellence.

www.cambridge.org
Information on this title: www.cambridge.org/9781009462587

DOI: 10.1017/9781009309578

First published 2023

A catalogue record for this publication is available from the British Library.

ISBN 978-1-009-46258-7 Hardback
ISBN 978-1-009-30958-5 Paperback
ISSN 2754-2912 (online)
ISSN 2754-2904 (print)

Cambridge University Press & Assessment has no responsibility for the persistence
or accuracy of URLs for external or third-party internet websites referred to in this
publication and does not guarantee that any content on such websites is, or will
remain, accurate or appropriate.

Every effort has been made in preparing this Element to provide accurate and up-to-date information
that is in accord with accepted standards and practice at the time of publication. Although case
histories are drawn from actual cases, every effort has been made to disguise the identities of the
individuals involved. Nevertheless, the authors, editors, and publishers can make no warranties that
the information contained herein is totally free from error, not least because clinical standards are
constantly changing through research and regulation. The authors, editors, and publishers therefore
disclaim all liability for direct or consequential damages resulting from the use of material contained
in this Element. Readers are strongly advised to pay careful attention to information provided by the
manufacturer of any drugs or equipment that they plan to use.

Governance and Leadership

Elements of Improving Quality and Safety in Healthcare

DOI: 10.1017/9781009309578
First published online: November 2023

Naomi J. Fulop and Angus I. G. Ramsay
Department of Applied Health Research, University College London

Author for correspondence: Naomi J. Fulop, n.fulop@ucl.ac.uk

Abstract: Lessons from service and system failures describe the pivotal roles played by governance and leadership in delivering high-quality, safe care. This Element sets out what the terms governance and leadership mean and how thinking about them has developed over time. Using real-world examples, the authors analyse research evidence on the influence of governance and leadership on quality and safety in healthcare at different levels in the health system: macro level (what national health systems do), meso level (what organisations do), and micro level (what teams and individuals do). The authors describe behaviours that may help boards focus on improving quality and show how different leadership approaches may contribute to delivering major system change. The Element presents some critiques of governance and leadership, including some challenges that can arise and gaps in the evidence, and then draws out lessons for those seeking to strengthen governance and leadership for improvement. This title is also available as Open Access on Cambridge Core.

Keywords: leadership, governance, accountability, performance management, engagement

ISBNs: 9781009462587 (HB), 9781009309585 (PB), 9781009309578 (OC)
ISSNs: 2754-2912 (online), 2754-2904 (print)

Contents

1 Introduction

Governance and leadership play a key role in delivering high-quality, safe care. In this Element, we set out what is meant by *governance* and *leadership*, discussing the way thinking has developed over time. We describe the role of governance and leadership in quality and safety at different levels, from the team or individual level to national policy. We discuss board governance, performance management, the influence of leadership on improvement efforts, and team-based leadership. Finally, we draw out lessons for practice, policy, and research, noting particular strengths and weaknesses in the evidence and what this means for governing and leading for quality and safety in healthcare settings in the future.

2 Why Are Governance and Leadership Important to Healthcare Quality and Safety?

We begin by outlining the role of governance and leadership in quality and safety (Section 2.1) and show that they can operate at multiple levels (Section 2.2), before we then go on to examine how governance and leadership might be defined and explain how thinking has evolved over time (Section 3).

2.1 The Role of Governance and Leadership in Quality and Safety

The central role played by governance and leadership in the actions (and inactions) relating to quality of care and patient safety has been repeatedly identified by inquiries and investigations into major organisational failures.[1] For instance, the 2002 inquiry into paediatric heart surgery at Bristol Royal Infirmary in the 1980s and 1990s[2] (also discussed in the Elements on statistical process control[3] and making culture change happen[4]) identified that there had been insufficient prioritisation and monitoring of quality, as well as a culture that failed to acknowledge problems. The recommendations of the Bristol inquiry were a key driver for the subsequent development of clinical governance ('inter-related activities aimed at improving the quality and safety of health care'[5]), which remains an important component of healthcare quality in the UK National Health Service (NHS).[1,2,5–7]

Despite efforts to improve care after the Bristol inquiry, problems have recurred. Investigations into higher-than-expected death rates at Mid Staffordshire NHS Foundation Trust in the late 2000s identified multiple failures of governance and leadership throughout the organisation and the wider system. These included the failure to monitor and enforce standards, insufficient transparency and involvement of patients and the public, and gaps in regional and national leadership.[1,8,9] More recently (2015), an investigation into serious incidents in Morecambe Bay maternity services found that poor processes for learning from adverse events, deficient clinical skills, and inadequate team-working contributed to the organisation's failure to maintain standards, which in turn resulted in serious incidents, including the deaths of mothers and babies.[10]

These inquiries and other investigations have consistently identified that organisational and system failures result from a combination of many inter-related factors. They also show that governance and leadership – through their influence on priorities, oversight, and management and culture – are often part of both problem and solution.

2.2 Governance and Leadership at Macro, Meso, and Micro Levels

Governance and leadership of healthcare operate at several levels. Here, we distinguish between macro (national), meso (organisational), and micro (team or individual) levels (see Figure 1).[11,12]

- In some systems, macro-level governance sets overarching direction and priorities for quality and safety (e.g. national recommendations), and may feature a variety of bodies serving different functions, including regulatory roles.[9,10,13]

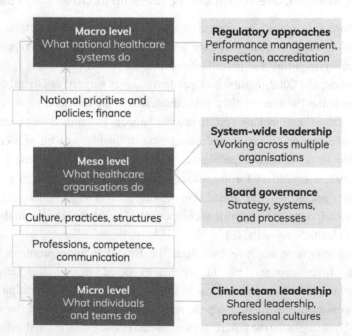

Figure 1 Governance at macro, meso, and micro levels with reference to examples discussed in this Element

The figure draws on work by Fulop and Ramsay.[11]

- At the meso level, organisations develop and implement strategies aimed at delivering high-quality, safe care to the populations they serve.
- Finally, at the micro level, frontline staff deliver this care.

These layers are heavily intertwined, with many points where different levels of governance and leadership interact. For example, at the macro (national/regional) level, a range of bodies may set policies, issue guidance, allocate resources, and operate incentives. Regulators may set standards and put mechanisms in place to oversee them and take action where needed.[14] At the meso (organisational) level, board governance may seek both to influence upwards into national priorities and to influence within their own organisations, and to bridge national drivers and frontline activity.[12,15] Understanding the interactions between these macro, meso, and micro levels is an important part of understanding how the quality and safety of care can be maintained and improved. In Figure 1, we describe these levels, some key processes, and where the examples selected for discussion in this Element sit in relation to these levels.

3 A Brief History

This section will discuss how thinking about governance and leadership has changed over time. It begins by setting out how the concepts have been defined, and the relationship between the two concepts. It then addresses how thinking about governance and leadership has evolved over the twentieth century to today.

3.1 What Is Meant by Governance and Leadership?

Governance and leadership are overlapping concepts with a complex relationship. Governance has been described as an 'elusive concept to define'.[16] The term derives from Latin words for 'to steer' or 'give direction'.[17] Its current meaning might be explained as follows:

- the means for achieving direction, control, and coordination of wholly or partially autonomous individuals or organisational units on behalf of interests to which they jointly contribute[18]
- ways in which organisations and the people working in them relate to each other[19]
- a set of processes (customs, policies, or laws) that are formally or informally applied to distribute responsibility or accountability among actors of a given [health] system.[16]

Therefore, governance may be seen in terms of the structures and processes that enable oversight, monitoring, and accountability within that system; but it is also important to note that any formal processes and structures may be shaped by (and should accommodate) the informal interactions between people operating within that system.

Leadership also tends to attract multiple definitions, but it can perhaps be summarised in terms of processes by which individuals or groups are enabled, encouraged, or inspired to achieve agreed goals within a given context. A common theme across various definitions is 'mobilising individuals, organisations and networks to formulate and/or enact purposes, values and actions which aim or claim to create valued outcomes for the public sphere'.[20]

There are important overlaps between the concepts of governance and leadership, for example, in terms of the aim to influence how people operate within a system or service. However, while the concepts overlap, they play different (yet interlinked) roles. That is, governance is a system that enables oversight, monitoring, and accountability of the processes and people operating within it; leadership may be seen as a key component of a governance system, acting both to influence and facilitate that system (e.g. shaping strategic vision and objectives, and enabling engagement with system processes).

3.2 How Has Thinking about Governance Changed?

Approaches to and thinking about governance in healthcare changed during the twentieth century and into the twenty-first century, reflecting broader social and political changes.[19] Traditionally, some healthcare professionals (e.g. doctors) operated forms of professional self-governance, in that they worked independently to deliver care while also gaining direction through their peer networks – for example, via the General Medical Council, established to regulate doctors in 1858,[21] and the General Nursing Council, established in 1919.[22]

Bureaucratic hierarchies emerged in the early to mid-twentieth century, characterised by a centralised authority implementing structures and rules in order to exert influence across the entire system. A key example was the hierarchical command and control approach of the NHS from its post-war inception. This system was led by a minister of government and the state department (the current equivalents being the Secretary of State for Health and Social Care and the Department of Health and Social Care, respectively) exerting influence through layers of authority all the way through to frontline delivery of care. The approach reflected the *big government* thinking that shaped the welfare state in the UK in the mid-twentieth century; it was embodied in the suggestion of Nye Bevan, the minister who oversaw the creation of the NHS, that 'when a bedpan is dropped on a hospital floor its noise should resound in the Palace of Westminster'.[23]

The command and control approach to running the NHS broadly continued until the 1980s when many nations, including the UK, parts of mainland

Europe, and New Zealand, began to adopt principles of market forces. This so-called *new public management* approach has been associated with the emergence of the 'new right' (e.g. the conservative movements led by Margaret Thatcher in the UK and Ronald Reagan in the USA in the 1980s). Drawing on private sector thinking to reshape approaches to running public services, including healthcare,[24] common features included:

- reduced centralised, hierarchical control accompanied by more corporate approaches to governance and management were introduced (e.g. introducing board governance)
- a purchaser–provider split and competitive tendering to deliver services
- a move from professional self-regulation to external audit and regulatory governance.[24]

Policy-makers anticipated that these changes would lead to greater entrepreneurialism and better quality care.[23] In practice, however, some research suggests that the shift to new public management may have been associated with reduced professional engagement, local democratic influence, and creative central policy-making, as well as depleting local capacity to balance long-term and short-term priorities.[24]

Since the early 2000s, the concept of *network governance* has grown in prominence as a possible way of enhancing collaboration between organisations while also engaging more effectively with a wider range of stakeholders, including the public, the voluntary sector, and frontline staff.[19,25,26] It may take a variety of forms,[25] with an important example the introduction of managed clinical networks for cancer services, which sought to assist in delivering the NHS national cancer plan.[27–29]

In practice, many health systems do not reflect different forms of governance in a pure sense, but rather in combination. For example, the current English NHS is characterised by overlapping features of markets (e.g. the purchaser–provider split) and network governance.[25] At the same time, bureaucratic governance (e.g. the enduring hierarchical influence of the Department of Health and Social Care and NHS England and Improvement[19,30]) and external regulation (e.g. operated by bodies such as the Care Quality Commission [CQC] and professional regulators[30–32]) are both highly consequential for the ways in which organisations providing care design and operate their own systems for governance and their leadership behaviours.

3.3 How Has Thinking about Leadership Changed?

Traditionally, thinking around leadership focused on the idea of *born leaders* and explored how individuals drew on their inherent qualities to lead others – the heroic leadership model.[33,34] Over the course of the last century, the focus shifted to characteristics commonly possessed by leaders (known as trait theory), and how leaders acted (behavioural theory). Contingency theory, which emerged in the 1950s, moved the focus to the relationship between leaders, their actions, and the organisational and wider contexts in which they operate.[35] Since the 2000s, research has increasingly addressed how leadership accommodates complexity within teams, organisations, and the wider system.[36,37] That is, individuals, groups, or organisations within a given setting may hold different and sometimes competing priorities, even when they are working towards a shared goal of improving quality and safety of care.

Researchers have also drawn a distinction between leadership strategies: 'transactional' strategies involve use of rewards and punishment to motivate, whereas 'transformational' strategies involve use of charisma, challenge, and individual focus to win others' trust and emotional buy-in to drive improvements.[38] Further, there has been a shift in perception from *leader as commander* to *leader as engager*, where leaders stimulate more collective approaches to leading on improvement.[39]

Understanding of *who* it is that leads has also changed over time. At microservice level, different staff groups have traditionally held different leadership responsibilities. For example, doctors tended to hold greater autonomy to influence practice and guide improvement than nurses.[40] But with the development of new public management in the 1980s, power shifted from professionals to managers as boards came to set priorities and facilitate improvement.[24] This seminal change was initially prompted by the Griffiths review into NHS management (1983), which reported that the NHS was unclear on objectives, performance, and quality, with little sense of who was in charge.[41–43] However, there is now growing recognition of the value of having a strong clinical voice in senior management.[44,45] This has led to development of 'hybrid' leaders who combine clinical and managerial roles and so may influence improvement both formally and informally.[46,47]

There have also been attempts to move beyond models of heroic individuals to consider models of shared leadership.[40,48] 'Distributed', 'shared', or 'collective' leadership proposes that leadership does not sit with one individual; rather, it encompasses anyone in an organisation or system who has a role in leading or managing activity – this includes middle management and frontline staff.[48–51] There is some evidence that high-performing healthcare organisations and clinical teams are more likely to feature aspects of shared leadership, while also retaining clear strategic direction from the top.[52,53] However, as we discuss later (Section 5.1), the effectiveness of distributed leadership may be influenced by context; for example, there are likely to be particular challenges when attempting to implement distributed leadership across complex systems that cover multiple organisations and sectors.[48,54]

4 Approaches in Action

In this section, we present evidence on how governance and leadership influence quality and safety. While we discuss evidence on governance and leadership separately, the two issues are closely intertwined. Section 4.1 describes how aspects of governance influence quality and safety. Sections 4.2 and 4.3 explore how board governance helps improve quality and safety, and the relationship between performance measurement, performance management, and regulation. Section 4.4 discusses leadership's contributions to quality and safety at macro, meso, and micro levels. Sections 4.5 and 4.6 illustrate these relationships in terms of leading major system change and how team leadership influences quality and safety.

4.1 How Does Governance Influence Quality and Safety?

The challenge of steering organisations and individuals to improve quality and safety can be framed in a number of ways.[53] For example, agency theory suggests the task is to develop systems and processes that manage individuals' self-interest,[53–56] whereas stewardship theory assumes individuals are all working towards the same goal and that the task of governance is more facilitative.[53,56,57] But whatever the conceptual model, governance typically involves setting strategy, ensuring accountability, and fostering an appropriate culture,[56,58] as outlined below.

4.1.1 Setting Strategy

Setting a long-term strategy refers to an overarching plan that describes how the organisation's values and priorities are to be achieved. It is important that strategy is linked to clear and measurable quality goals. National policies or standards at system level typically frame the context in which healthcare organisations operate and the priorities they seek to achieve.[11,59] Closer to the front line, organisational strategies for quality set the tone for staff and teams, while also framing the objectives against which performance is measured (e.g. see Section 4.2 on contributions of board governance to quality and safety).[12,50,54,58–60]

4.1.2 Ensuring Accountability

Effective systems of accountability – monitoring and measuring performance, perhaps linked to meaningful incentives – are critical elements of governance of a quality strategy. At the macro level, such systems are visible in national regulation and inspection processes.[11,20] Within organisations, boards may develop and implement local audit and clinical governance processes.[43,50,59,61–64]

4.1.3 Fostering Culture

Shaping *culture* (the 'shared aspects of organisational life'[65]) has a vital part to play in ensuring that long-term strategies and systems of accountability can work most effectively. Cultures that explicitly prioritise characteristic features of high-quality care delivery (for example, commitment to improvement, patient experience, engagement, and teamwork) are thought to support better care.[50,59,66] However, a review of the evidence cautions that conventional assessments of organisational culture are often too simplistic, since organisations are often home to a multitude of cultures at the micro level. Further, the interrelationships between organisational culture and improving quality and safety are likely to be complex; for example, culture may influence different improvement activities differently, and the culture itself might be shaped by how an organisation delivers on quality.[65] Further discussion of some of the issues relating to culture can be found in the Element on making culture change happen.[4]

4.2 How Board-Level Governance Can Contribute to Improving Quality and Safety

We have already identified three important governance roles for boards: setting strategy, ensuring accountability, and fostering culture. In this section, we discuss how boards enact their governance roles to support delivery of high-quality, safe care, presenting evidence on how boards interact with both the organisations they govern and their wider context.[45,55,60,64,69,70]

'Board governance' refers to the systems and processes used by senior leadership in healthcare organisations to support delivery of key organisational priorities, including high-quality, safe care.[45,55,60] Boards are accountable for the quality and safety of care in the organisations they lead.[45,55,60,71] But these are not boards' only priorities; others include, for example, resource management, finances, innovation, population health, workforce, and equality and diversity. To govern effectively, boards must achieve an appropriate balance between all these priorities.[60,72]

What boards do and how they do it is important to the quality and safety of care that their organisations provide.[1,45,55,73] Evidence from the USA and the UK suggests that boards tend to perform better on quality and safety if they make quality a strategic priority, dedicate time to discussing quality in board meetings, and establish dedicated quality committees.[52,60,70,74,75] In the following sections, we discuss some of the ways in which boards can strengthen their focus on quality.

4.2.1 Using Strategy to Drive Quality

A key role of boards is to set the strategy for the organisation they lead. Quality should be at the heart of this strategy.[60,72] Research on boards in Australia has identified the importance of translating broad strategic statements into specific, meaningful quality objectives, since, in the absence of such statements, board members and staff struggled to discuss progress on improvement.[76]

An analysis of the approaches used by English boards to enable quality improvement (QI) used an evidence-based measure that reflected the degree to which boards prioritise, understand, engage with, and support QI – referred to as QI 'maturity'. This study indicated the importance of both the amount of time dedicated to quality *and* its focus. Boards of organisations with high QI maturity spent the bulk of their time discussing quality and prioritising issues that had been escalated by the quality committee, trusting the wider governance structure to identify the issues that required attention.[45]

4.2.2 Engaging Stakeholders at All Levels to Build Cultures that Prioritise Quality

Boards that are effective at leading improvement achieve it by engaging stakeholders at macro, meso, and micro levels (reflecting their accountability to different levels of the system) and translating this engagement into strategic priorities.[77-79] Such boards seek to manage their wider environment – including regulators, payer organisations (commonly described as commissioners in the English NHS), and fellow provider organisations – in order to support region-wide responses to quality challenges. Equally, they may engage with local stakeholders to build cultures that are supportive of improvement, patient engagement, and teamwork.[52,60,80-82] For example, boards of the organisations judged to have high QI maturity were found to engage actively with stakeholders, including clinicians and patient groups, so that different stakeholders could help shape organisational priorities for quality.[45]

4.2.3 Using Data to Ensure Accountability and Drive Improvement

Boards that are successful in focusing on quality make use of data to drive improvement, rather than just for external assurance.[45,61] They do this by clearly defining what is meant by quality and endorsing its associated measures. They create and regularly review a quality monitoring framework, analyse performance against benchmarks over time to identify areas of improvement, and assess progress on areas of concern.[1,45] Drawing on a combination of hard quantitative data on performance and soft data (e.g. discussions with clinicians or patients, or walk-arounds by senior management) has been found to help boards understand the realities of quality and safety on the ground and to help make a compelling case for improvement.[45,64,73,83,84]

4.2.4 Communication and Information to Support Understanding and Prioritisation of Quality

Effective communication about quality at board level – for example, presenting clear narratives on quality while being open to questioning and challenge – can help offer board members the space to reflect on the reasons for any quality and safety issues, and potential solutions.[85] Also important is the capacity to use, interpret, and act on available data. Boards of Australian organisations with low engagement with quality described themselves as 'drowning in data',[45] while English boards with low QI maturity received data that made it 'hard to see the wood from the trees'.[85] Boards with high QI maturity, on the other hand, outlined the use of benchmarks linked directly with improvement priorities[45] and managers created a logical narrative through the data, thereby facilitating rapid understanding and better engagement from board members.[85] Boards with high QI maturity highlighted the advantages of effective challenge (e.g. questioning assumptions behind analyses and actions) in creating a wider understanding of quality issues across the board.[45,85] They also set in place communication systems that aimed to support shared understanding of quality issues across departments and professions at every level.[45,78,86]

4.2.5 What Helps Boards Govern for Quality?

Boards can be helped to carry out their governance roles by ensuring they have the appropriate membership and that board members continue to develop their capabilities in relation to quality. Board membership needs to be sufficiently large and sufficiently diverse to provide the necessary expertise to govern complex healthcare organisations.[60,64] For instance, research on healthcare organisations in the UK, USA, and elsewhere suggests that a higher proportion of doctors on boards has been associated with better performance on quality ratings and patient outcomes.[87–89] This may be because clinicians offer greater understanding of quality and safety, and communicate more effectively with clinical staff.[69,87,88] However, how these clinicians behave also matters: boards with high QI maturity included clinicians who were assertive and vocal on matters of quality; less mature organisations had fewer such members.[45] The balance of executive management and non-executive (lay) members is also important.[72] Non-executives, ideally with expertise in quality and safety, provide a valuable perspective in scrutinising performance – challenging senior management on quality and safety and how they are balanced against other organisational priorities.[55]

Boards that address quality effectively prioritise learning and development.[80,81,83,90] They learn from external examples of good practice to drive initial improvement, then analyse local problem-solving to develop tailored improvement strategies.[45,80] Members of these boards are also more likely to have undergone formal QI training – for example, on what quality means and relevant improvement techniques, including investigation (e.g. root cause analysis) and improvement approaches (e.g. plan-do-study-act cycles).[45] Board-level improvement tools can support the development of effective organisational QI strategies and at a relatively low cost, but support from senior board members is necessary for such interventions to have optimal impact.[91]

4.3 The Role of Performance Measurement and Performance Management in Improving Quality and Safety

In this section, we discuss how performance measurement and performance management have been used in an effort to strengthen accountability for healthcare quality and safety.[12,92–94] Internationally, demand for accountability for healthcare quality and safety is growing.[95] Performance measurement (judging how a service performs against targets) has increased in prominence as a tool of accountability in health and other sectors since the late 1970s, with the first national performance indicators implemented in the NHS in 1983.[96] Alongside this, performance management (the techniques and approaches used to create or shape performance) has also become more prominent.[96]

Performance measurement and performance management differ in important ways. Measurement involves collecting and comparing data on how organisations are doing – for instance, in complying with quality standards (e.g. in a national audit) or on delivery of outcomes (e.g. infection or mortality rates). By contrast, performance management entails an active response to measurement of how organisations are doing in order to drive improved performance.[97] For instance, many health systems, including in the USA (Medicare), the EU, and the UK, incentivise provision of high-quality, safe care.[1,95]

We now discuss how different aspects of performance measurement and management influence quality and safety, and some associated pitfalls.

4.3.1 Performance Measurement

Performance measures may help communicate priorities, while targets seek to define what constitutes good and bad levels of performance on a given measure.[94,96] Targets may support significant improvements in processes associated with quality of care. For instance, the introduction of national targets and monitoring for healthcare-associated infection (such as methicillin-resistant

Staphylococcus aureus [MRSA] and *Clostridium difficile*) was associated with an increase in hospitals' governance and improvement activity on this issue.[98] Similarly, national thresholds for time taken to see patients were associated with pronounced reductions in patient waiting times.[99,100]

However, targets can have several downsides. They may lead to box-ticking, where staff do enough to achieve the target in ways that do not reflect its spirit. For example, in response to a 5-minute waiting-time target intended to encourage rapid patient triage in emergency rooms, hospitals introduced 'hello nurses' who greeted patients quickly but did little else. So the target was met but without achieving the intended benefit.[92] A further potential downside in target-driven regimes is that what is measured becomes what matters. This may mean that important but harder-to-measure aspects of care (such as the humanity of care) are overlooked.

Sometimes target-setting may thwart the goals it is intended to serve or cause confusion of purpose. For example, error reporting has an important role to play in understanding patient safety, but the message it presents is complex, as a higher number of reported errors may reflect a stronger focus on patient safety.[101–103] This challenge can be observed in the context of medication errors, which are substantially under-reported; this makes it difficult to set a target to reduce error, which in turn may have contributed to reduced focus on governing this important safety issue.[98]

The range of techniques used to assess performance is wide, and each can have positive and negative effects: there is no single right answer. For example, self-measurement – where an organisation or service measures and reports its own performance – can be performed rapidly but runs the risk of 'fiddling' the figures (distorting or even falsifying data).[92,96]

4.3.2 Responses to Performance Management

Responses to performance management are mixed. For example, publishing performance data and incentivising performance through financial penalties or rewards (as described in Box 1) can help to drive improvements in quality and safety.[104] But they can also have unintended consequences. One consequence of performance management is that it can reduce the 'slack' – the space to think and act – available to boards, thereby limiting their capacity to develop their improvement strategies.[105] Other examples include reduced appetite to take on high-risk cases[106,107] and increased risk of gaming targets, such as ratchet effects, where services seek to improve only slightly on the previous year's performance (e.g. on waiting times), permitting a perception of ongoing progress at the expense of the patients who might benefit from larger and more immediate improvements in quality.[92,94,96]

> ### Box 1 Financial incentives for performance
>
> The relationship between financial incentives and performance has been explored in several studies. Research on hospitals in north-west England found that while pay for performance was associated with initial reductions in patient mortality,[108] this effect was not sustained long term.[109] Research on US hospitals has also indicated no significant effect of financial incentives on patient mortality,[110] and research on payment for performance in primary care in England has reported similarly limited effect on quality and outcomes of care.[111,112] A review of qualitative research on primary care in England suggests that while pay for performance activity fitted well with clinicians' desire for personal success, it clashed with their prioritisation of self-direction, benevolence, and creativity; the review recommended that gaining clinicians' acceptance of any definition of 'high-quality care' would be key to achieving greater engagement with such schemes.[113]

4.4 How Does Leadership Influence Quality and Safety?

Given that its goals include influencing and mobilising, leadership has the potential to encourage and facilitate improvement (and the cultures associated with improvement) at every level.

- At the macro level, leadership sets the tone for a whole system, framing national and regional priorities, driving engagement in systems of accountability, and encouraging intraregional initiatives and interregional learning.[20,114]
- At the meso level, leadership (e.g. boards) defines the vision for an organisation and engages local staff in improvement activity, while also reaching out to external organisations to shape region-wide endeavours.[40,52,56,60,66]
- And at the micro level, frontline leadership helps ensure clinical teams work together to improve quality and safety, while responding to rapid changes in circumstance.[40,53,90]

Effective leadership for quality and safety requires clear understanding of priorities, both in terms of external drivers and local issues. In order to be able to identify such issues and the appropriate responses, research suggests that leaders will benefit not only from expertise and experience in improving quality and safety,[115,116] but also the humility to recognise that change might be needed in one's own services.[44,116,117]

Providing clarity about goals and priorities – defining and stating the purpose of action and change – is important for communicating why improvement is necessary.[20,40,118,119] Doing so consistently and clearly may help people to understand the desirability of the prioritised action and behaviours.[40,115,116,119,120]

Being able to engage and enable others is a key element of leadership for quality and safety. Bringing about improvement requires commitment across a wide range of stakeholders, some of whom might not accept that change is required. Leaders therefore need to embody integrity and fairness, and take a consistent approach in order to inspire commitment to improvement. It is similarly important that both leaders and those they are leading have the capabilities and capacity to participate in such activities.[40,45,66,90,115,117,119]

Though 'heroic' leadership is a discredited approach, leaders' personal characteristics and capabilities may play a role in how effective they are at influencing others. The evidence identifies experience, technical expertise, extraversion, and conscientiousness as important characteristics.[121] Political skill and awareness are also increasingly seen as important facilitators of leading improvement.[20,114] How a leader relates to and is seen by teams is critical. The perceived status of different professional groups matters, too. Evidence from health and care settings shows that staff prefer to be led by a fellow professional, placing trust in their expertise and understanding. However, it is those from 'higher status' professions, such as doctors, who tend to gain leadership roles.[48,54] Traditional hierarchies in healthcare settings can make it harder for leaders from professions that have tended to be denied high status, such as nursing, to be seen as legitimate leaders.

4.5 Understanding How Leadership Influences Major System Change

In this section, we discuss how leadership influences major system change, including reorganisation of specialist care across multiple healthcare organisations at regional level.[35] Major system change has been linked with better care and outcomes (e.g. improvements in mortality or length of hospital stay).[122–127] But such change is complex, often taking many years and substantial effort to plan and implement, and it requires sustained collaboration with multiple stakeholders in contrasting situations and with conflicting priorities.[51] System change may be controversial, prompting resistance from local leaders, clinicians, and the wider public.

As we discuss, different forms of leadership play important roles in delivering major system change, addressing both the challenges of complex change and associated resistance. Bottom-up clinical leadership can help to ensure suitably designed systems that are supported by the people who will deliver them; top-down, region-wide leadership can encourage relevant stakeholders not to withdraw from discussions in the change process. Some of the key approaches that can contribute to the success of major system change are outlined below.

4.5.1 Engaging and Collaborating with the Right Stakeholders

Leading major system change relies on engaging and working in collaboration with the right stakeholders. As major system change commonly addresses a whole patient pathway across a region, multiple different groups may contribute in different ways. For example, clinicians – including primary care, hospital specialist services, and ambulance services – are vital to ensuring services deliver appropriate care and that patients are transferred reliably.[128–130] Major system change is also unlikely to happen unless it has backing in terms of resources and governance from payer organisations (commissioning organisations in the context of the English NHS) and senior hospital management.[130] Further, major system change should reflect the needs of patients and the public; this means engaging them and their representatives, including charities and politicians. Common examples of engagement activities include consultation (e.g. through distributing public surveys about proposals and holding open meetings where members of the public may raise questions or concerns) or involving stakeholders in planning and oversight groups.[131]

Given that these different stakeholders may have competing priorities, a key leadership challenge is keeping stakeholders on board throughout the change process – from the initial agreement to change, through planning and implementation, to ongoing sustainability of the new system. A common challenge to major system change relates to concerns about the loss of local services or activity; this may come from clinicians, healthcare organisations, or local communities.

4.5.2 Combining Top-Down and Bottom-Up Approaches

Box 2 details two examples of the reorganisation of stroke services in London and Greater Manchester that provide an interesting exploration of top-down and bottom-up leadership approaches.

4.5.3 Leading Implementation of a Provider Network

Provider networks – where provider organisations (e.g. NHS acute trusts) collaborate formally to deliver a particular care pathway – are another option for delivering major system change.[25] An example of successful leadership in implementing a provider network, London Cancer, is described in Box 3.

One critique of the leadership approaches used in major system change argues that leaders may use clinical arguments politically to sideline the voice of local (clinical and public) stakeholders who are against change.[133]

BOX 2 TOP-DOWN AND BOTTOM-UP LEADERSHIP APPROACHES IN A MAJOR SYSTEM CHANGE OF STROKE SERVICES

London's major system change of stroke services combined top-down and bottom-up leadership. Change was led by the London Strategic Health Authority (top-down), which worked with clinical leaders (stroke and ambulance services) across the region to design the new system. Strong clinical (bottom-up) leadership shaped the objectives and design of the new services and undertook a substantial public consultation exercise. Combining top-down authority with bottom-up clinical engagement resulted in system-wide ownership of the changes, which helped to overcome local resistance to the proposals.[130,132]

In contrast, Greater Manchester's changes were mainly bottom-up, led by the local stroke network. The network was highly effective at bringing stakeholders on board. However, they hit difficulties when some local services threatened to withdraw from the change process upon learning that they might lose activity under the proposed changes. To keep these organisations on board, the network adapted the service model by altering the eligibility criteria for treatment in a specialist unit. This meant that all hospitals continued to treat some stroke patients. But although local hospitals stayed engaged, the less radical service model did not lead to significant improvements in care delivery and outcomes, as had been achieved through London's changes.[124,125,130]

In the absence of region-wide authority, other leadership approaches have been observed. For example, Greater Manchester centralised their stroke services further in 2015, following a long period of delay. One factor that made a difference was the introduction of top-down leadership through the launch of a region-wide board in late 2014. The new board included leaders of clinical commissioning groups[*] and hospitals, and the board drove rapid system-wide agreement of changes, completed in spring 2015. This new system resulted in significant improvements in care and outcomes across the region.[123,125]

---

[*] Clinical commissioning groups were a form of payer organisation. They were introduced in 2013 following a major reorganisation of the governance of the NHS in England, and were replaced in 2022 by integrated care boards.

Box 3 Establishing a provider network to implement a major system change of specialist cancer surgical services

London Cancer, a network of provider organisations, was established to implement a major system change of specialist cancer surgical services across a geographical footprint covering a population of 3.2 million.[128]

Research on the network's implementation of a major system change for urological and oesophagogastric cancers identified several processes that supported delivery of change. These included:

- a consistent core leadership team (made up of senior clinicians with enhanced leadership skills)
- sharing responsibility with clinicians and managers across different levels of the system (facilitated by experienced network managers)
- engaging actively with key stakeholders.

Consistent core leadership: the chief medical officer (a clinician from a separate, non-surgical specialty) and the network board (chaired by a cancer survivor and made up of experts based outside London) led the programme. Local clinicians and managers felt the chief medical officer and network board offered strong, objective leadership, which helped enable support for the changes.

Sharing responsibility at multiple levels: for each clinical pathway that was to be centralised, a pathway lead working within that specialty was appointed. Pathway leads chaired committees whose membership comprised other local clinicians operating within that clinical pathway. Together, they were responsible for leading development and delivery of the new services, which in turn enabled greater ownership of the proposed changes within local services.

Engaging stakeholders: cancer survivors (and patient representative groups) were directly involved in governance at every level of the programme, including as members of the overall programme board and cancer pathway-specific boards. This approach improved patient engagement and facilitated wider public involvement. In addition, when new payer organisations were established (see Box 2), leaders of London Cancer engaged with them actively. This helped to ensure that the major system change process underwent appropriate scrutiny and was supported by payer organisations and providers across the local system.[128]

Equally, such critiques may underplay the extent to which this resistance is driven by professional and organisational vested interests, which may not coincide with the interests of patients and the public; an important example of this is the (understandable) desire of clinicians and managers to resist changes that might disadvantage their own services (e.g. through loss of specialist activity resulting in fewer training opportunities and loss of attractiveness to medical trainees).[125,130,134,135]

4.6 How Does Team Leadership Influence Quality and Safety?

Delivering safe, high-quality care relies on effective collaboration between highly specialised professionals.[53,136,137] Effective teamwork is associated with better performance on quality and safety,[136–138] including lower mortality, fewer patient safety incidents, and better staff well-being and retention.[136,139–141] In contrast, teams that do not work well together are less likely to deliver high-quality care.[61,137,139] In this section, we outline how leadership works at team or micro level.[142]

Effective teams tend to have shared quality objectives; they have inclusive approaches to decision-making, information sharing, conflict management, and learning, with an underlying engaging and supportive team leadership.[68,137,139] Leadership is frequently identified as central to fostering team cultures and behaviours that support high-quality, safe care.[53,136,137] This includes the creation of psychological safety, whereby team members feel that they can raise questions or share concerns or fears with their colleagues. (Further discussion of psychological safety can be found in the Element on workplace conditions.[143])

One useful way of thinking about team leadership is to consider its focus – first on the people in the team, and second on the tasks to be achieved[144] – as discussed in the next two sections.

4.6.1 Person-Focused Leadership

Person-focused leadership involves engaging and inspiring team members to work together. To do this, leaders communicate both their vision for quality and their confidence that the team can achieve it. Leading by example – for instance, demonstrating consistent commitment to high standards – may encourage a shared approach to delivering care.[144]

Enabling shared leadership, where responsibility is distributed across team members in line with their (professional or patient-specific) expertise, is thought to be associated with more effective decision-making.[53,136,144] By focusing on team members individually, understanding their aspirations, and providing

Box 4 Person-focused team leadership in community-based care

Research on integrated community-based health and social care teams in England has shown that team leadership approaches may make important differences to how teams operate and deliver high-quality care.[136,144] These teams developed through a national initiative (the NHS vanguard programme)[145] that sought to integrate health and social care in the community and reduce pressures on hospital services.

The research drew on a review of the literature and qualitative research with staff based in 10 community interprofessional teams. In particular, staff discussed how person-focused aspects of team leadership contributed to effective teamwork and service-user outcomes. Several important examples are set out below.

- **Motivating the team:** team leaders who maintained a positive attitude, communicating confidence in the team's abilities to deliver on its vision and objectives, were seen as more able to sustain team morale during difficult periods.
- **Walking the talk:** setting high standards and being seen to embody these consistently, and demonstrating authority if required, were viewed as important in building team members' confidence in their ability to deliver on their goals.
- **Collaborative learning and improvement:** team members reported the value of prioritising improvement of their service and being enabled to work together to agree objectives for or approaches to change. Creating safe spaces where staff could raise concerns and propose solutions was seen as important for developing plans that fitted the context and were owned by team members.
- **Considering individuals:** recognising and working with individual needs was seen as key to developing the team overall while ensuring its individual members felt valued. Examples of this included team leaders viewing each team member as an individual, providing constructive feedback, and tailoring development to reflect personal aspirations while also complementing the team's objectives.
- **Empowering staff:** sharing responsibility – for example, for decision-making – across the team was reported as being important for developing teamwork. At the same time, by providing advice or assuming responsibility for higher risk actions, team leaders supported the autonomy of individual staff ('letting us get on with it') and enabled staff to deal with problems directly.

- **Team building and maintenance:** a team approach was taken in both day-to-day activities (e.g. by managing group dynamics to ensure all voices were heard, or creating clear and consistent boundaries for team member roles) and formal and informal team exercises (e.g. team-based development activities or social events).
- **Emotional intelligence:** staff referred to the importance of empathy, communication, and openness to help staff feel valued and understood and to promote healthy communication across the team.

constructive feedback, leaders are able to make staff feel valued, confident, and more part of the team (see Box 4).[144]

Supporting the team in discussing, learning, and collaborating around quality appears to result in better problem-solving and a stronger sense of team membership and common goals.[136,144] This is supported further by creating a clear sense of team identity and purpose.[136,144] For example, research on mental health teams has indicated the importance of having team leaders who can chair team meetings effectively. When team leaders were able to create a space for the team to agree key care decisions, share ideas, and work through disagreements constructively, this set the tone for the team.[141]

The task of team leadership may become more complex when teams cover more than one profession or sector. Staff in integrated teams reflected that health and social care have different leadership cultures: social care is less hierarchical than healthcare and has more formalised mechanisms of support for staff.[144]

4.6.2 Task-Focused Leadership

Task-focused leadership relates to the processes by which team goals are achieved. Having a shared sense of objectives, responsibilities, and delivery helps to ensure that all team members are working to achieve the same quality goals; and, as goals become clearer, so does team effectiveness.[116,136,137,144] Next, building expertise (e.g. by addressing gaps in knowledge or skills and enabling access to training) increases the team's capabilities to deliver high-quality care.[116,136,144] Then, leading beyond the team, in order to promote it with stakeholders within and beyond the organisation, can improve access to shared resources (e.g. diagnostics) and help to build wider networks across local systems.[116,136,144,146]

Underlying these processes are team leaders' personal qualities: in addition to expertise and focus on quality and innovation,[136] they bring enthusiasm, empathy, emotional intelligence, and communication skills.[136,144] Staff in integrated community teams highlighted the importance of a team leader who could 'walk the talk' and act as a role model for other members of the team, and they emphasised the importance of leaders who maintained a positive, constructive approach during difficult times.[144]

5 Critiques of Governance and Leadership

5.1 Navigating the Complex Challenges of Governance and Leadership

There is probably no single best way to govern or lead for improving quality and safety. The examples explored in this Element show that the effects of governance and leadership are strongly influenced by context at the macro, meso, and micro levels. Contingency theory suggests that different styles of governance may work better depending on circumstances. For example, inward-focused organisations (those that focus mainly on internal processes) may achieve greater staff commitment, while outward-looking organisations (those that prioritise the wider context, including neighbouring organisations, regulators, and policy-makers) might engage more effectively with external regimes.[67] Important influences include policy priorities and organisational challenges – factors that should not be seen in isolation but understood, rather, as highly interrelated.[20,40,116,120,147–149]

Earlier, we highlighted a number of unintended consequences of some approaches to governance, including the risks of reduced capacity to balance long-term and short-term priorities, reduced creativity in central policy-making (Section 3.2), and downsides associated with target-driven regimes (Section 4.3). We also showed that adapting approaches to healthcare governance from those used elsewhere – for example, importing thinking, structures, and processes from the business sector (Section 3.2) to inform new public management – is not straightforward. The question of stakeholders illustrates some of these complexities: while governance in the business sector relates to shareholders, the main stakeholder in a public health system could be said to be society in all its guises.[12,24,60,62] As a result, there are active debates about how to ensure democratic, public accountability[12,24] and how best to involve the public in making decisions about major changes to the organisation of care.[131,132] Closer to the micro level, the example of root cause analysis, a technique originally used to investigate incidents in industrial settings, further illustrates some of the challenges of transferring learning into healthcare. In industrial settings, root cause analysis operates as a learning technique and prioritises the avoidance of blame. In healthcare settings, however, root cause analysis may take on additional functions of establishing responsibility for an incident and extending organisational surveillance and control; this in turn reduces the envisaged learning benefits.[150]

Similarly, though considerable efforts have been made to improve approaches to regulation (Box 5), research on the CQC's influence on performance describes how regulators may be feared by the organisations they regulate.[151] Fearfulness can prompt organisations to become closed and defensive, which in turn limits the effectiveness of regulatory activity. NHS

BOX 5 DEVELOPMENT OF THE CQC'S INSPECTION APPROACH

In 2013, the CQC introduced a new approach to inspection, which included more precisely targeted care standards and extended site visits conducted by larger, more expert teams.[151] Research on this approach described the important relationship between inspectors and local staff: inspectors needed to be sufficiently skilled and experienced to be perceived as credible and sufficiently consistent to be trusted; local teams needed to be willing to discuss improvement openly. A key challenge identified for inspectors was the need to build a close and supportive relationship with healthcare teams, while also maintaining sufficient objectivity.[151]

In 2014, the CQC extended its inspection approach to dig further into leadership of organisations[152] and, in so doing, suggested that the priorities of a 'well-led' organisation should be:

• setting a clear vision for the organisation
• having clear governance and accountability processes
• fostering a culture that is transparent and quality-focused
• engaging with both staff and patients
• learning and finding new ways to improve.

From 2021, following experiences of the COVID-19 pandemic, the CQC adapted their approach to inspection further.[153,154] On-site service inspections would no longer be conducted routinely; instead, they would happen only when there was a clear need for them, for instance when there were clear signs of a change in quality of care, or where necessary information was unavailable. In support of this more risk-based approach, CQC emphasised the importance of both hard and soft intelligence, including enhanced routine data monitoring, and strengthened communication with services and members of the wider community. From 2022, CQC began a staged introduction of a new single assessment framework.[155] This aimed to simplify the regulation process and to link assessment more closely to stakeholder priorities, guided by new quality statements ('We statements'), shaped by public expectations of services.

England's special measures regime for improving quality (which operated from 2014 to 2021, when it was replaced with the Recovery Support Programme)[156] provides a recent illustration of the potential impact of macro-level performance management on organisations.[44] Under this regime, organisations rated by the CQC as 'inadequate' on leadership and other qualities entered special measures for quality, a process that included an offer of external support and oversight to improve quality.[44,151] Organisations also required support to mitigate the emotional cost and stigma associated with being placed in special measures. Further, improving performance from a low starting point required substantial additional resources, both in terms of the time required to make change (2–3 years) and sustainable funding for long enough to result in improved performance.[44]

None of this is to say that regulation and governance are bad things, but it does emphasise the need for optimised design and execution. According to Smithson et al., a constructive, quality-focused relationship between regulators and those regulated is more likely to result in positive experiences of regulation and improvements in healthcare quality.[151] Considering regulation as a 'social process' means that both regulators and those regulated may contribute to more productive interactions, characterised by longstanding relationships, openness, mutual trust and respect, shared values and agreed ways of working, opportunities to interact informally, and experienced and respected inspectors who possess the interpersonal skills to conduct inspection with consistency and fairness.[151]

The challenges of leadership are similarly complex. Whether leading at board level[45,116] or within a clinical team,[119] effective leadership relies in part on assessing and responding to present and oncoming shifts in context. Making sense of these complex and dynamic changes in context is likely to play an important part in effective leadership for quality.[20] Of course, that requires the right approach to leadership. As discussed earlier (Section 3.3), much thinking on leadership has traditionally drawn on what are now fairly outdated understandings of how leadership works – for instance, the focus on heroic models, which contrasts with the reality that achieving high-quality care is likely to rely on more collective efforts. Since the early 2000s, there has been a shift to seeing distributed leadership as an effective way to encourage creative innovations at the frontline.[48–50,90,157] But distributed leadership (where leadership is spread though different levels of an organisation or system) is not in itself a panacea: while effective healthcare does rely on drawing together expertise from a range of disciplines,[53,136,137] researchers have also noted that managerial and professional hierarchies may simultaneously work against attempts to share leadership.[48,54]

Governance and leadership across sectors can be particularly challenging when leadership is also shared – with a risk that such distributed leadership becomes fractured in practice.[48] Frontline staff and local leaders may have a clear view of how to deliver high-quality care within their own team, but their views may be influenced by a desire to protect their services from change. As illustrated by the two examples of stroke service reorganisation (see Box 2), these vested interests may have to be challenged to improve care quality.[11,45,83]

Accelerated by the COVID-19 pandemic, recent thinking has proposed 'the need for public sector transformations to support the robust governance of turbulence'.[158] It is argued that many traditional approaches to governance are not fit to address turbulent, disruptive challenges, especially in an era of rapid technological advances where information and other resources may be transferred quickly across the world, and where the nature of problems to be addressed is unclear. Discussions of governance during this period,[158] supported by a literature review of public service responses to the turbulence prompted by COVID-19,[159] suggest that robustness can be achieved through agile network governance, where public organisations meet new challenges creatively in close partnership with the private sector and wider society. This work identifies seven strategies that characterise governance for turbulence:[159]

- scalability – where resources may be increased or decreased to support responses to immediate and changing demands
- prototyping – iterative development of innovative solutions, based on evaluation of rapid feedback
- modularisation – where multiple solutions are developed in parallel to address separate components of a developing situation
- bounded autonomy – building local and regional ownership of a strategy, drawing together system leaders, service providers, and members of the public
- bricolage – making creative and adaptive use of available resources to fashion a response when no tailored response exists
- strategic polyvalence – where solutions are designed so that they might serve multiple strategic purposes
- voluntary compliance – importantly, evidence on responses to COVID-19 suggested that robustness of governance responses to turbulence rely on co-creation between public organisations and consenting members of the public.

Important priorities for governing in turbulent times include active engagement with frontline staff and external experts, a willingness to work with incomplete or uncertain data, distribution of responsibility to actors best suited to an emerging problem, willingness to experiment and an acceptance of the risk of associate failure, and enhanced communication with all stakeholders.[158]

5.2 Gaps in the Evidence

Some clear gaps and challenges in the evidence remain. Although much has been written about how governance and leadership could or should work, we are still learning about their relationship with quality and safety. In particular, much remains to be understood about which aspects of governance and leadership result in better quality, how they exert that influence, and under which circumstances. In part, this relates to a number of limitations in how we think about governance and leadership, and how their relationship with quality and safety has been analysed to date.

First, there are some important challenges in relation to how governance and leadership are defined and understood. As outlined in Section 3.1, different definitions of both concepts have emerged, raising questions about the extent to which research is addressing the same thing. Examples of such difficulties include terms like 'leadership' and 'management' being used interchangeably,[39] and supposedly contrasting leadership approaches being applied in very similar ways in practice.[120]

Second, there are limitations in terms of the type of evidence that has been generated. The overall quality of the evidence base for the impact of governance and leadership on performance has been questioned.[48] Further, in many cases the direction of the relationship may be uncertain; for example, high performance might *enable* certain governance or leadership approaches, rather than be the result of them. While some researchers propose that randomised controlled trials (RCTs) are required to better understand the impact of governance and leadership on aspects of quality and safety,[160] RCT-type evidence is unlikely to be appropriate for understanding many of the phenomena presented here. This is because many of the factors that RCTs seek to control for (e.g. organisational context and interactions with it) in fact play a pivotal role in how governance and leadership work in practice. Excluding these factors limits the value of such analyses.[161] Some research has shown associations between certain approaches to governance and leadership and performance on quality,[74,75,87] and other research acknowledges how different approaches play out in different contexts.[68]

Studies that account for the integral role of context are likely to provide many useful lessons about *how* governance and leadership contribute to quality and safety – for example, approaches making use of qualitative and quantitative methods, process evaluations, and in-depth ethnographic studies are likely to be valuable.[162–164] Longitudinal, theory-driven research of this kind can help open up this black box to explain how governance and leadership influence quality and safety. We have highlighted several examples of such research in this Element, but more are needed; given the powerful influence of context there is a clear need for further research to be conducted in a range of settings. As research funders continue to prioritise such work, we anticipate that understanding of these complex relationships will continue to grow over the coming years.

6 Conclusions

This Element has analysed how governance and leadership shape and influence organisation and delivery of healthcare quality and safety at macro, meso, and micro levels of the system. Governance and leadership may contribute both to significant improvements and major failures in delivering high-quality, safe care, so it is important to get them right. We have described conditions that might help to ensure that performance measures, targets, and regulatory activities support rather than hinder organisations in improving quality (e.g. aligned targets, sufficient organisational capacity). We have outlined behaviours that may help boards focus more effectively on improving quality (e.g. prioritisation of quality, focused discussions informed by a range of hard and soft data, engaging stakeholders both within and beyond the organisation). We have also set out how different leadership approaches contribute to delivering major system change (e.g. how combining top-down authority and bottom-up clinical leadership can help sustain stakeholder participation and challenge local vested interests). Finally, we have shown how person-centred and team-centred leadership may influence the ways in which teams work together to deliver high-quality, safe care (e.g. effective chairing of meetings may support a greater shared sense of purpose, while engaging with and valuing team members as individuals may help build psychological safety). Box 6 provides a summary of the lessons that can be drawn from the evidence.

> BOX 6 LESSONS ON HOW GOVERNANCE AND LEADERSHIP INFLUENCE QUALITY
> AND SAFETY AT MACRO, MESO, AND MICRO LEVELS
>
> **At Macro Level (National)**
>
> - Incentives (e.g. targets, payments) can encourage implementation and sustainability of change, but they may also have unintended consequences (e.g. gaming targets). Those who manage, deliver, and use services therefore need to contribute to the development of the objectives associated with these incentives to ensure buy-in.
> - Interventions to support struggling organisations may support improvements in quality but may also introduce significant practical and emotional burdens. Resources are needed to ensure that organisations have the skills and capacity to develop and deliver an improvement strategy.
>
> **At Meso Level (Systems and Organisations)**
>
> - Quality and safety need to be a central priority for board activity. That means inclusion on agendas, creating systems to support understanding of quality, and dedicating resources to build expertise in quality.
> - To build a compelling case for improving quality, board and divisional leaders should draw on a range of both hard data and soft data (e.g. patient narratives). A central challenge is to then engage key stakeholder groups (including staff, patients, and carers) to build a shared understanding of quality and a culture that is supportive of quality. For example, this can be achieved by leaders attending stakeholder events, inviting stakeholders to board meetings, and visiting various care settings.
> - Board development and self-assessment tools (e.g. on QI maturity) may help boards to adopt processes that are more effective in addressing quality and, in turn, develop more successful organisational improvement strategies.
> - Boards may also look beyond their own organisation – for example, learning from improvement approaches used in neighbouring organisations, or by contributing to system-wide improvement activities.
> - Implementing system-level improvements is complex and may be facilitated by combining top-down and bottom-up leadership approaches.
>
> **At Micro Level (Clinical Teams)**
>
> - Person-centred leadership includes focusing on team members' individual needs and aspirations, and providing constructive feedback and development opportunities. Such actions may improve the team's

overall skill mix and help to ensure that team members feel valued, thereby increasing their sense of belonging and ownership of team priorities.

- Taking a task-centred approach may also support quality. Creating shared objectives and responsibility for quality across the team is central to shaping a culture that is supportive of improvement. Using established team processes (e.g. routine discussions of clinical cases, team away-days, training or coaching sessions) to facilitate decision-making, learning, and collaboration around quality and safety can help to achieve this. It may also enhance team members' psychological safety, thereby encouraging open discussions about improvement and increasing innovation. However, achieving or maintaining a shared culture across teams may become more challenging as membership becomes more diverse and complex.

7 Further Reading

Defining Governance and Leadership

- Davies et al.[19] – a review that describes the history and mechanisms of different modes of governance.
- Ferlie et al.[18] – an overview of thinking about macro, meso, and micro levels in health systems.
- Hartley and Benington[38] – an overview of approaches to leadership in healthcare.
- Øvretveit[40] – a review of how governance and leadership influence quality.

Influencing Improvement through Governance and Leadership

- Braithwaite[90] – an analysis of factors influencing QI.
- Fulop and Ramsay[11] – an analysis of how organisations influence quality and safety.
- McKean and Snyderman[116] – a review of leadership's influence on safety, drawing on healthcare and other sectors.
- Mannion and Davies[67] – an analysis of the influence of context and culture on quality in care, with a focus on governance.

Performance Measurement and Management

- Pollitt[96] – a literature review of performance management over the past 40 years.
- Mannion and Braithwaite[92] – a review identifying the pitfalls of performance measurement in the English NHS.
- Smithson et al.[151] – an evaluation of the CQC's approach to inspecting health and social care providers.

Leadership of Major System Change

- Best et al.[51] – a literature review describing factors influencing large system transformation, including leadership.
- Turner et al.[130] – a qualitative analysis of leadership approaches used in a major system change of acute stroke services in London and Greater Manchester.
- Vindrola-Padros et al.[128] – a qualitative analysis of leadership approaches used by a provider network in implementing a major system change of specialist cancer surgical services.
- Fraser et al.[133] – an editorial drawing on research evidence, presenting a critique of approaches to leading major system change.

Board Governance

- Chambers et al.[55,165] – a literature review[55] and qualitative study[165] of board governance, including membership and dynamics.
- Jones et al.[45] – a mixed-methods study of how boards operate in healthcare organisations with high and low QI maturity.

Team Leadership

- Aufegger et al.[53] – a review of the literature on how shared leadership might contribute to effectiveness of clinical team management.
- Smith et al.[144] – an article drawing together a review of the evidence and qualitative research on the contribution of leadership to teamwork and effectiveness in community health and social care teams.

Contributors

Both authors contributed to conceptualisation of this Element, the selection and interpretation of evidence presented, and drafting of the Element at all stages of its development. Both authors have approved the final version, and agree to be accountable for all aspects of the work in ensuring that questions related to its accuracy or integrity are appropriately investigated and resolved.

Conflicts of Interest

Naomi J. Fulop is a non-executive director on the board of Whittington Health NHS Trust.

Acknowledgements

We thank the peer reviewers and editorial team for their insightful comments and recommendations to improve the Element. A list of peer reviewers is published at www.cambridge.org/IQ-peer-reviewers. Naomi J. Fulop is a National Institute for Health Research (NIHR) Senior Investigator. The views and opinions expressed in this Element are those of the authors and do not necessarily reflect those of the NIHR, NHS, or the Department of Health and Social Care.

Funding

This Element was funded by THIS Institute (The Healthcare Improvement Studies Institute, www.thisinstitute.cam.ac.uk). THIS Institute is strengthening the evidence base for improving the quality and safety of healthcare. THIS Institute is supported by a grant to the University of Cambridge from the Health Foundation – an independent charity committed to bringing about better health and healthcare for people in the UK.

About the Authors

Naomi J. Fulop is Professor of Health Care Organisation and Management in the Department of Applied Health Research, University College London. Her research interests are at the interface between health policy and delivering, managing, and organising healthcare services.

Angus I. G. Ramsay is Principal Research Fellow in the Department of Applied Health Research, University College London. He is interested in using mixed-method evaluation approaches to understand how organisational factors influence efforts to improve quality of care and patient outcomes.

Creative Commons License

References

1. Brown A, Dickinson H, Kelaher M. Governing the quality and safety of healthcare: A conceptual framework. *Soc Sci Med* 2018; 202: 99–107. https://doi.org/10.1016/j.socscimed.2018.02.020.

2. Kennedy I. *The Report of the Public Inquiry into Children's Heart Surgery at the Bristol Royal Infirmary 1984–1995: Learning from Bristol*. London: The Stationery Office; 2002. https://psnet.ahrq.gov/issue/learning-bristol-report-public-inquiry-childrens-heart-surgery-bristol-royal-infirmary-1984 (accessed 22 May 2023).

3. Mohammed MA. Statistical process control. In: Dixon-Woods M, Brown K, Marjanovic S, et al., eds. *Elements of Improving Quality and Safety in Healthcare*. Cambridge: Cambridge University Press; forthcoming.

4. Mannion R. Making culture change happen. In: Dixon-Woods M, Brown K, Marjanovic S, et al., eds. *Elements of Improving Quality and Safety in Healthcare*. Cambridge: Cambridge University Press; 2022. https://doi.org/10.1017/9781009236935.

5. Travaglia JF, Debono D, Spigelman AD, Braithwaite J. Clinical governance: A review of key concepts in the literature. *Clin Gov* 2011; 16: 62–77. https://doi.org/10.1108/14777271111104592.

6. Walshe K, Offen N. A very public failure: Lessons for quality improvement in healthcare organisations from the Bristol Royal Infirmary. *BMJ Qual Saf* 2001; 10: 250–6. https://doi.org/10.1136/qhc.0100250.

7. Public Health England. Newborn hearing screening programme (NHSP) operational guidance. *Clinical Governance*. www.gov.uk/government/publications/newborn-hearing-screening-programme-nhsp-operational-guidance/4-clinical-governance (accessed 22 May 2023).

8. Francis R. *Independent Inquiry into Care Provided by Mid Staffordshire NHS Foundation Trust January 2005–March 2009*. London: The Stationery Office; 2010. www.gov.uk/government/publications/independent-inquiry-into-care-provided-by-mid-staffordshire-nhs-foundation-trust-january-2001-to-march-2009 (accessed 22 May 2023).

9. Francis R. *Report of the Mid Staffordshire NHS Foundation Trust Public Inquiry*. London: The Stationery Office; 2013. www.gov.uk/government/publications/report-of-the-mid-staffordshire-nhs-foundation-trust-public-inquiry (accessed 22 May 2023).

10. Kirkup B. *The Report of the Morecambe Bay Investigation: An Independent Investigation into the Management, Delivery and Outcomes of Care Provided*

by the Maternity and Neonatal Services at the University Hospitals of Morecambe Bay NHS Foundation Trust from January 2004 to June 2013. London: The Stationery Office; 2015. www.gov.uk/government/publications/ morecambe-bay-investigation-report (accessed 22 May 2023).

11. Fulop NJ, Ramsay AIG. How organisations contribute to improving the quality of healthcare. *BMJ* 2019; 365: l1773. https://doi.org/10.1136/bmj .l1773.

12. Ferlie E, Baeza JI, Addicott R, Mistry R. The governance of pluralist health care systems: An initial review and typology. *Health Serv Manage Res* 2017; 30: 61–71. https://doi.org/10.1177/0951484816682395.

13. Department of Health. *High Quality Care for All: NHS Next Stage Review Final Report*. London: Department of Health; 2008. https://assets .publishing.service.gov.uk/government/uploads/system/uploads/attach ment_data/file/228836/7432.pdf (accessed 22 May 2023).

14. Walshe K. The rise of regulation in the NHS. *BMJ* 2002; 324: 967–70. https://doi.org/10.1136/bmj.324.7343.967.

15. Lipunga AM, Tchereni BM, Bakuwa RC. Emerging structural models for governance of public hospitals. *Int J Health Gov* 2019; 24: 98–116. https:// doi.org/10.1108/IJHG-03-2019-0018.

16. Barbazza E, Tello JE. A review of health governance: Definitions, dimensions and tools to govern. *Health Policy* 2014; 116: 1–11. https://doi.org/10 .1016/j.healthpol.2014.01.007.

17. Cornforth C, Chambers N. *The Role of Corporate Governance and Boards in Organisational Performance*. Cambridge: Cambridge University Press; 2010. http://oro.open.ac.uk/23907/5/Chapter_on_governance_boards_ and_performance_020709.pdf (accessed 22 May 2023).

18. Lynn Jr LE, Heinrich CJ, Hill CJ. *Improving Governance: A New Logic for Empirical Research*. Washington, DC: Georgetown University Press; 2001.

19. Davies C, Anand P, Artigas L, et al. *Links between Governance, Incentives and Outcomes: A Review of the Literature*. London: National Co-ordinating Centre for NHS Service Delivery and Organisation R&D; 2005. https://njl-admin.nihr.ac.uk/document/download/2008497 (accessed 22 May 2023).

20. Hartley J. Ten propositions about public leadership. *Int J Public Leadersh* 2018; 14: 202–17. https://doi.org/10.1108/IJPL-09-2018-0048.

21. Irvine D. A short history of the General Medical Council. *Med Educ* 2006; 40: 202–11. https://doi.org/10.1111/j.1365-2929.2006.02397.x.

22. Bradshaw A. Competence and British nursing: A view from history. *J Clin Nurs* 2000; 9: 321–9. https://doi.org/10.1046/j.1365-2702.2000.00399.x.

23. Exworthy M, Powell M, Mohan J. Markets, bureaucracy and public management: The NHS: Quasi-market, quasi-hierarchy and quasi-network?

Public Money Manag 1999; 19: 15–22. https://doi.org/10.1111/1467-9302.00184.

24. Ferlie E. The new public management and public management studies. In: Aldag R, ed. *Oxford Research Encyclopedia of Business Management.* New York: Oxford University Press; 2017. https://doi.org/10.1093/acrefore/9780190224851.013.129.

25. Provan KG, Kenis P. Modes of network governance: Structure, management, and effectiveness. *J Public Adm Res Theory* 2008; 18: 229–52. https://doi.org/10.1093/jopart/mum015.

26. Caffrey L, Ferlie E, McKevitt C. The strange resilience of new public management: The case of medical research in the UK's National Health Service. *Public Adm Rev* 2019; 21: 537–58. https://doi.org/10.1080/14719037.2018.1503702.

27. Addicott R, McGivern G, Ferlie E. The distortion of a managerial technique? The case of clinical networks in UK health care. *Br J Manag* 2007; 18: 93–105. https://doi.org/10.1111/j.1467-8551.2006.00494.x.

28. Addicott R, Ferlie E. Understanding power relationships in health care networks. *J Health Organ Manage* 2007; 21: 393–405. https://doi.org/10.1108/14777260710778925.

29. Ferlie E, McGivern G, Fitzgerald L. A new mode of organizing in health care? Governmentality and managed networks in cancer services in England. *Soc Sci Med* 2012; 74: 340–7. https://doi.org/10.1016/j.socscimed.2011.03.021.

30. Osipovič D, Allen P, Sanderson M, Moran V, Checkland K. The regulation of competition and procurement in the National Health Service 2015–2018: Enduring hierarchical control and the limits of juridification. *Health Econ Policy Law* 2020; 15: 308–24. https://doi.org/10.1017/S1744133119000240.

31. Kjaer PF, Vetterlein A. Regulatory governance: Rules, resistance and responsibility. *Contemp Politics* 2018; 24: 497–506. https://doi.org/10.1080/13569775.2018.1452527.

32. Beaussier A-L, Demeritt D, Griffiths A, Rothstein H. Accounting for failure: Risk-based regulation and the problems of ensuring healthcare quality in the NHS. *Health Risk Soc* 2016; 18: 205–24. https://doi.org/10.1080/13698575.2016.1192585.

33. Stogdill RM. Leadership, membership and organization. *Psychol Bull* 1950; 47: 1–14. https://doi.org/10.1037/h0053857.

34. Wood M. The fallacy of misplaced leadership. *J Manage Stud* 2005; 42: 1101–21. https://doi.org/10.1111/j.1467-6486.2005.00535.x.

35. Kumar RD. Leadership in healthcare. *Anaesth Intensive Care Med* 2013; 14: 39–41. https://doi.org/10.1016/j.mpaic.2012.11.006.

36. Belrhiti Z, Giralt AN, Marchal B. Complex leadership in healthcare: A scoping review. *Int J Health Policy Manage* 2018; 7(12): 1073–84. www .ncbi.nlm.nih.gov/pmc/articles/PMC6358662/ (accessed 22 May 2023).

37. Plsek PE, Wilson T. Complexity, leadership, and management in healthcare organisations. *BMJ* 2001; 323(7315): 746–9. www.bmj.com/content/323/ 7315/746.1.short (accessed 22 May 2023).

38. Hartley J, Benington J. *Leadership for Healthcare*. Bristol: Policy Press; 2010.

39. Reichenpfader U, Carlfjord S, Nilsen P. Leadership in evidence-based practice: A systematic review. *Leadersh Health Serv* 2015; 28: 298–316. https://doi.org/10.1108/LHS-08-2014-0061.

40. Øvretveit J. *Leading Improvement Effectively: Review of Research*. London: The Health Foundation; 2009. www.health.org.uk/publications/ leading-improvement-effectively (accessed 22 May 2023).

41. Griffiths R. *NHS Management Inquiry*. London: Department of Health and Social Security; 1983. www.sochealth.co.uk/national-health-service/grif fiths-report-october-1983 (accessed 22 May 2023).

42. Klein R. The National Health Service (NHS) at 70: Bevan's double-edged legacy. *Health Econ Policy Law* 2019; 14: 1–10. https://doi.org/10.1017 /S1744133117000354.

43. Gorsky M. 'Searching for the people in charge': Appraising the 1983 Griffiths NHS Management Inquiry. *Med Hist* 2013; 57: 87–107. https://doi .org/10.1017/mdh.2012.82.

44. Vindrola-Padros C, Ledger J, Hill M, et al. The special measures for quality and challenged provider regimes in the English NHS: A rapid evaluation of a national improvement initiative for failing healthcare organisations. *Int J Health Policy Manag* 2022; 11(12): 2917. https://doi.org/10.34172/ ijhpm.2022.6619.

45. Jones L, Pomeroy L, Robert G, et al. How do hospital boards govern for quality improvement? A mixed methods study of 15 organisations in England. *BMJ Qual Saf* 2017; 26: 978–86. https://doi.org/10.1136/bmjqs-2016-006433.

46. Waring J. Restratification, hybridity and professional elites: Questions of power, identity and relational contingency at the points of 'professional–organisational intersection'. *Sociol Compass* 2014; 8: 688–704. https://doi .org/10.1111/soc4.12178.

47. Currie G, Burgess N, Hayton JC. HR practices and knowledge brokering by hybrid middle managers in hospital settings: The influence of professional

hierarchy. *Hum Resour Manage* 2015; 54: 793–812. https://doi.org/10
.1002/hrm.21709.

48. Currie G, Lockett A. Distributing leadership in health and social care: Concertive, conjoint or collective? *Int J Manage Rev* 2011; 13: 286–300. https://doi.org/10.1111/j.1468-2370.2011.00308.x.

49. Gronn P. Distributed leadership as a unit of analysis. *Leadersh Q* 2002; 13: 423–51. https://doi.org/10.1016/S1048-9843(02)00120-0.

50. Bolden R. Distributed leadership in organizations: A review of theory and research. *Int J Manage Rev* 2011; 13: 251–69. https://doi.org/10.1111/j
.1468-2370.2011.00306.x.

51. Best A, Greenhalgh T, Lewis S, et al. Large-system transformation in health care: A realist review. *Milbank Q* 2012; 90: 421–26. https://doi.org/10.1111
/j.1468-0009.2012.00670.x.

52. Baker GR. *The Roles of Leaders in High-Performing Health Care Systems*. London: The King's Fund; 2011. www.kingsfund.org.uk/sites/default/files/ roles-of-leaders-high-performing-health-care-systems-ross-baker-kings-fund-may-2011.pdf (accessed 22 May 2023).

53. Aufegger L, Shariq O, Bicknell C, Ashrafian H, Darzi A. Can shared leadership enhance clinical team management? A systematic review. *Leadersh Health Serv* 2019; 32: 309–35. https://doi.org/10.1108/LHS-06-2018-0033.

54. Currie G, Spyridonidis D. Sharing leadership for diffusion of innovation in professionalized settings. *Hum Relations* 2019; 72: 1209–33. https://doi .org/10.1177/0018726718796175.

55. Chambers N, Harvey G, Mannion R. Who should serve on health care boards? What should they do and how should they behave? A fresh look at the literature and the evidence. *Cogent Bus Manage* 2017; 4: 1–14. https:// doi.org/10.1080/23311975.2017.1357348.

56. Bennington L. Review of the corporate and healthcare governance literature. *J Manage Organ* 2010; 16: 314–33. https://doi.org/10.5172/jmo .16.2.314.

57. Eeckloo K, Delesie L, Vleugels A. Where is the pilot? The changing shapes of governance in the European hospital sector. *J R Soc Promot Health* 2007; 127: 78–86. https://doi.org/10.1177/1466424007075457.

58. Chambers N, Harvey G, Mannion R, Bond J, Marshall J. Towards a framework for enhancing the performance of NHS boards: A synthesis of the evidence about board governance, board effectiveness and board development. *Health Serv Deliv Res* 2013; 1: 6. https://doi.org/10.3310/hsdr01060.

59. Thiel A, Winter V, Büchner VA. Board characteristics, governance objectives, and hospital performance: An empirical analysis of German hospitals.

Health Care Manage Rev 2018; 43: 282–92. https://doi.org/10.1097/HMR .0000000000000153.

60. Ramsay AIG, Fulop N, Fresko A, Rubenstein S. *The Healthy NHS Board: Review of Guidance and Research Evidence.* Leeds: NHS Leadership Academy; 2013. www.yumpu.com/en/document/view/39165116/healthy-nhs-board-a-review-of-nhs-leadership-academy (accessed 22 May 2023).

61. Dixon-Woods M, Baker R, Charles K, et al. Culture and behaviour in the English National Health Service: Overview of lessons from a large multi-method study. *BMJ Qual Saf* 2014; 23: 106–15. https://doi.org/10.1136/bmjqs-2013-001947.

62. Chambers N. Healthcare board governance. *J Health Organ Manage* 2012; 26: 6–14. https://doi.org/10.1108/14777261211211133.

63. Baker GR, Denis J-L, Pomey M-P, MacIntosh-Murray A. Designing effective governance for quality and safety in Canadian healthcare. *Healthc Q* 2010; 13: 38–45. https://doi.org/10.12927/hcq.2013.21244.

64. Mannion R, Davies H, Freeman T, et al. Overseeing oversight: Governance of quality and safety by hospital boards in the English NHS. *J Health Serv Res Policy* 2015; 20: 9–16. https://doi.org/10.1177/1355819614558471.

65. Mannion R, Freeman T, Millar R, Davies H. Effective board governance of safe care: A (theoretically underpinned) cross-sectioned examination of the breadth and depth of relationships through national quantitative surveys and in-depth qualitative case studies. *Health Serv Deliv Res* 2016; 4: 4. https://doi.org/10.3310/hsdr04040.

66. Parand A, Dopson S, Renz A, Vincent C. The role of hospital managers in quality and patient safety: A systematic review. *BMJ Open* 2014; 4: e005055. https://doi.org/10.1136/bmjopen-2014-005055.

67. Mannion R, Davies H. Understanding organisational culture for healthcare quality improvement. *BMJ* 2018; 363: k4907. https://doi.org/10.1136/bmj .k4907.

68. West MA, Lyubovnikova J, Eckert R, Denis J-L. Collective leadership for cultures of high quality health care. *J Organ Eff People Perf* 2014; 1: 240–60. https://doi.org/10.1108/JOEPP-07-2014-0039.

69. Millar R, Mannion R, Freeman T, Davies HT. Hospital board oversight of quality and patient safety: A narrative review and synthesis of recent empirical research. *Milbank Q* 2013; 91: 738–70. https://doi.org/10.1111 /1468-0009.12032.

70. Martin GP, Aveling E-L, Campbell A, et al. Making soft intelligence hard: A multi-site qualitative study of challenges relating to voice about safety concerns. *BMJ Qual Saf* 2018; 27: 710–7. https://doi.org/10.1136/ bmjqs-2017-007579.

71. Freeman T, Millar R, Mannion R, Davies H. Enacting corporate governance of healthcare safety and quality: A dramaturgy of hospital boards in England. *Sociol Health Illn* 2016; 38: 233–51. https://doi.org/10.1111/1467-9566 .12309.

72. Ramsay AIG, Fulop N, Fresko A, Rubenstein S. *The Healthy NHS Board: A Review of Guidance and Research Evidence*. London: Department of Health; 2010. www.leadershipacademy.nhs.uk/wp-content/uploads/2013/ 06/NHSLeadership-HealthyNHSBoard-2010-LiteratureReview.pdf (accessed 22 May 2023).

73. Tsai TC, Jha AK, Gawande AA, et al. Hospital board and management practices are strongly related to hospital performance on clinical quality metrics. *Health Aff* 2015; 34: 1304–11. https://doi.org/10.1377/hlthaff .2014.1282.

74. Jha A, Epstein A. Hospital governance and the quality of care. *Health Aff* 2010; 29: 182–7. https://doi.org/10.1377/hlthaff.2009.0297.

75. Jha AK, Epstein AM. A survey of board chairs of English hospitals shows greater attention to quality of care than among their US counterparts. *Health Aff* 2013; 32: 677–85. https://doi.org/10.1377/hlthaff.2012.1060.

76. Brown A. Understanding corporate governance of healthcare quality: A comparative case study of eight Australian public hospitals. *BMC Health Serv Res* 2019; 19: 725. https://doi.org/10.1186/s12913-019- 4593-0.

77. Bate P, Mendel P, Robert G. *Organizing for Quality: The Improvement Journeys of Leading Hospitals in Europe and the United States*. Abingdon: Radcliffe; 2007.

78. Care Quality Commission. *Quality Improvement in Hospital Trusts: Sharing Learning from Trusts on a Journey of QI*. London: Care Quality Commission; 2018. www.cqc.org.uk/publications/evaluation/quality- improvement-hospital-trusts-sharing-learning-trusts-journey-qi (accessed 22 May 2023).

79. Baker GR, MacIntosh-Murray A, Porcellato C, et al. *High Performing Healthcare Systems: Delivering Quality by Design*. Toronto: Longwoods; 2008. www.longwoods.com/publications/books/571/1/high-performing- healthcare-systems-delivering-quality-by-design (accessed 22 May 2023).

80. Nembhard IM, Cherian P, Bradley EH. Deliberate learning in health care: The effect of importing best practices and creative problem solving on hospital performance improvement. *Med Care Res Rev* 2014; 71: 450–71. https://doi.org/10.1177/1077558714536619.

81. Burnett S, Mendel P, Nunes F, et al. Using institutional theory to analyse hospital responses to external demands for finance and quality in five

European countries. *J Health Serv Res Policy* 2016; 21: 109–17. https://doi.org/10.1177/1355819615622655.

82. Damschroder LJ, Aron DC, Keith RE, et al. Fostering implementation of health services research findings into practice: A consolidated framework for advancing implementation science. *Implement Sci* 2009; 4: 50. https://doi.org/10.1186/1748-5908-4-50.

83. Dixon-Woods M, McNicol S, Martin G. Ten challenges in improving quality in healthcare: Lessons from the Health Foundation's programme evaluations and relevant literature. *BMJ Qual Saf* 2012; 21: 876–84. https://doi.org/10.1136/bmjqs-2011-000760.

84. Martin GP, McKee L, Dixon-Woods M. Beyond metrics? Utilizing 'soft intelligence' for healthcare quality and safety. *Soc Sci Med* 2015; 142: 19–26. https://doi.org/10.1016/j.socscimed.2015.07.027.

85. Brown A. Communication and leadership in healthcare quality governance: Findings from comparative case studies of eight public hospitals in Australia. *J Health Organ Manag* 2020; 34: 144–61. https://doi.org/10.1108/JHOM-07-2019-0194.

86. Curry LA, Spatz E, Cherlin E, et al. What distinguishes top-performing hospitals in acute myocardial infarction mortality rates? A qualitative study. *Ann Intern Med* 2011; 154: 384–90. https://doi.org/10.7326/0003-4819-154-6-201103150-00003.

87. Veronesi G, Kirkpatrick I, Vallascas F. Clinicians on the board: What difference does it make? *Soc Sci Med* 2013; 77: 147–55. https://doi.org/10.1016/j.socscimed.2012.11.019.

88. Sarto F, Veronesi G. Clinical leadership and hospital performance: Assessing the evidence base. *BMC Health Serv Res* 2016; 16: 169. https://doi.org/10.1186/s12913-016-1395-5.

89. Sarto F, Veronesi G, Kirkpatrick I. Organizing professionals and their impact on performance: The case of public health doctors in the Italian SSN. *Publ Manage Rev* 2019; 21: 1029–51. https://doi.org/10.1080/14719037.2018.1544270.

90. Braithwaite J. Changing how we think about healthcare improvement. *BMJ* 2018; 361: k2014. https://doi.org/10.1136/bmj.k2014.

91. Barbosa EC, Jones L, Pomeroy L, et al. A board level intervention to develop organisation-wide quality improvement strategies: Cost-consequences analysis in 15 healthcare organisations. *Int J Health Policy Manag* 2022; 11: 173–82. https://doi.org/10.34172/IJHPM.2020.91.

92. Mannion R, Braithwaite J. Unintended consequences of performance measurement in healthcare: 20 salutary lessons from the English National

Health Service. *Intern Med J* 2012; 42: 569–74. https://doi.org/10.1111/j .1445-5994.2012.02766.x.

93. Lapsley I. New public management: The cruellest invention of the human spirit? *Abacus* 2009; 45: 1–21. https://doi.org/10.1111/j.1467-6281 .2009.00275.x.

94. Bevan G, Hood C. What's measured is what matters: Targets and gaming in the English public health care system. *Public Adm* 2006; 84: 517–38. https://doi.org/10.1111/j.1467-9299.2006.00600.x.

95. Busse R, Klazinga N, Panteli D, Quentin W, eds. *Improving Healthcare Quality in Europe: Characteristics, Effectiveness and Implementation of Different Strategies.* Brussels: European Observatory on Health Systems and Policies; 2019. https://apps.who.int/iris/bitstream/handle/10665/ 327356/9789289051750-eng.pdf (accessed 22 May 2023).

96. Pollitt C. Performance management 40 years on: A review. Some key decisions and consequences. *Publ Money Manag* 2018; 38: 167–74. https://doi.org/10.1080/09540962.2017.1407129.

97. Lebas MJ. Performance measurement and performance management. *Int J Prod Econ* 1995; 41: 23–35. https://doi.org/10.1016/0925-5273(95) 00081-X.

98. Ramsay AIG, Magnusson C, Fulop N. The relationship between external and local governance systems: The case of health care associated infections and medication errors in one NHS trust. *Qual Saf Health Care* 2010; 19: e45. https://doi.org/10.1136/qshc.2009.037473.

99. Boyne GA, Chen AA. Performance targets and public service improvement. *J Publ Adm Res Theory* 2007; 17: 455–77. https://doi.org/ 10.1093/jopart/mul007.

100. Kelman S, Friedman JN. Performance improvement and performance dysfunction: An empirical examination of distortionary impacts of the emergency room wait-time target in the English National Health Service. *J Publ Adm Res Theory* 2009; 19: 917–46. https://doi.org/10.1093/jopart/mun028.

101. Reason J. Safety paradoxes and safety culture. *Inj Control Saf Promot* 2000; 7: 3–14. https://doi.org/10.1076/1566-0974(200003)7:1;1-V;FT003.

102. Weaver SJ, Lubomksi LH, Wilson RF, et al. Promoting a culture of safety as a patient safety strategy: A systematic review. *Ann Intern Med* 2013; 158: 369–74. https://doi.org/10.7326/0003-4819-158-5-201303051- 00002.

103. Braithwaite J, Westbrook MT, Travaglia JF, Hughes C. Cultural and associated enablers of, and barriers to, adverse incident reporting. *BMJ Qual Saf* 2010; 19: 229–33. https://doi.org/10.1136/qshc.2008.030213.

104. Campanella P, Vukovic V, Parente P, et al. The impact of public reporting on clinical outcomes: A systematic review and meta-analysis. *BMC Health Serv Res* 2016; 16: 296. https://doi.org/10.1186/s12913-016-1543-y.

105. Jones L, Pomeroy L, Robert G, et al. Explaining organisational responses to a board-level quality improvement intervention: Findings from an evaluation in six providers in the English National Health Service. *BMJ Qual Saf* 2019; 28: 198–204. https://doi.org/10.1136/bmjqs-2018-008291.

106. Behrendt K, Groene O. Mechanisms and effects of public reporting of surgeon outcomes: A systematic review of the literature. *Health Policy* 2016; 120: 1151–61. https://doi.org/10.1016/j.healthpol.2016.08.003.

107. Williams MP, Modgil V, Drake MJ, Keeley F. The effect of consultant outcome publication on surgeon behaviour: A systematic review and narrative synthesis. *Ann R Coll Surg Engl* 2018; 100: 428–35. https://doi.org/10.1308/rcsann.2018.0052.

108. Sutton M, Nikolova S, Boaden R, et al. Reduced mortality with hospital pay for performance in England. *N Engl J Med* 2012; 367: 1821–8. https://doi.org/10.1056/NEJMsa1114951.

109. Kristensen SR, Meacock R, Turner AJ, et al. Long-term effect of hospital pay for performance on mortality in England. *N Engl J Med* 2014; 371: 540–8. https://doi.org/10.1056/NEJMoa1400962.

110. Jha AK, Joynt KE, Orav EJ, Epstein AM. The long-term effect of premier pay for performance on patient outcomes. *N Engl J Med* 2012; 366: 1606–15. https://doi.org/10.1056/NEJMsa1112351.

111. Ryan AM, Krinsky S, Kontopantelis E, Doran T. Long-term evidence for the effect of pay-for-performance in primary care on mortality in the UK: A population study. *Lancet* 2016; 388: 268–74. https://doi.org/10.1016/S0140-6736(16)00276-2.

112. Harrison MJ, Dusheiko M, Sutton M, et al. Effect of a national primary care pay for performance scheme on emergency hospital admissions for ambulatory care sensitive conditions: Controlled longitudinal study. *BMJ* 2014; 349: g6423. https://doi.org/10.1136/bmj.g6423.

113. Khan N, Rudoler D, McDiarmid M, Peckham S. A pay for performance scheme in primary care: Meta-synthesis of qualitative studies on the provider experiences of the quality and outcomes framework in the UK. *BMC Fam Pract* 2020; 21: 142. https://doi.org/10.1186/s12875-020-01208-8.

114. Hartley J, Sancino A, Bennister M, Resodihardjo SL. Leadership for public value: Political astuteness as a conceptual link. *Publ Admin* 2019; 97: 239–49. https://doi.org/10.1111/padm.12597.

115. Alderwick H, Charles A, Jones B, Warburton W. *Making the Case for Quality Improvement: Lessons for NHS Boards and Leaders*. London: The King's Fund; 2017. www.kingsfund.org.uk/publications/making-case-quality-improvement (accessed 22 May 2023).

116. McKean EL, Snyderman CH. Leadership driving safety and quality. *Otolaryngol Clin North Am* 2019; 52: 11–22. https://doi.org/10.1016/j.otc.2018.08.002.

117. Kool M, van Dierendonck D. Servant leadership and commitment to change, the mediating role of justice and optimism. *J Organ Chang Manag* 2012; 25: 422–33. https://doi.org/10.1108/09534811211228139.

118. Kempster S, Jackson B, Conroy M. Leadership as purpose: Exploring the role of purpose in leadership practice. *Leadership* 2011; 7: 317–34. https://doi.org/10.1177/1742715011407384.

119. Künzle B, Kolbe M, Grote G. Ensuring patient safety through effective leadership behaviour: A literature review. *Saf Sci* 2010; 48: 1–17. https://doi.org/10.1016/j.ssci.2009.06.004.

120. Donovan S-L, Salmon PM, Lenné MG. Leading with style: A literature review of the influence of safety leadership on performance and outcomes. *Theor Issues Ergonomics Sci* 2016; 17: 423–42. https://doi.org/10.1080/1463922X.2016.1143986.

121. Caldwell C, Dixon RD, Floyd LA, et al. Transformative leadership: Achieving unparalleled excellence. *J Bus Ethics* 2012; 109: 175–87. https://doi.org/10.1007/s10551-011-1116-2.

122. Ramsay AIG, Morris S, Hoffman A, et al. Effects of centralizing acute stroke services on stroke care provision in two large metropolitan areas in England. *Stroke* 2015; 46: 2244–51. https://doi.org/10.1161/STROKEAHA.115.009723.

123. Morris S, Ramsay AIG, Boaden R, et al. Impact and sustainability of centralising acute stroke services in English metropolitan areas: Retrospective analysis of hospital episode statistics and stroke national audit data. *BMJ* 2019; 364: l1. https://doi.org/10.1136/bmj.l1.

124. Morris S, Hunter RM, Ramsay AIG, et al. Impact of centralising acute stroke services in English metropolitan areas on mortality and length of hospital stay: Difference-in-differences analysis. *BMJ* 2014; 349: g4757. https://doi.org/10.1136/bmj.g4757.

125. Fulop NJ, Ramsay AIG, Hunter RM, et al. Evaluation of reconfigurations of acute stroke services in different regions of England and lessons for implementation: A mixed-methods study. *Health Serv Deliv Res* 2019; 7: 7. https://doi.org/10.3310/hsdr07070.

126. Van den Heede K, Dubois C, Mistiaen P, et al. Evaluating the need to reform the organisation of care for major trauma patients in Belgium: An analysis of administrative databases. *Eur J Trauma Emerg Surg* 2019; 45: 885–92. https://doi.org/10.1007/s00068-018-0932-9.

127. Moran CG, Lecky F, Bouamra O, et al. Changing the system: Major trauma patients and their outcomes in the NHS (England) 2008–17. *eClinicalMedicine* 2018; 2: 13–21. https://doi.org/10.1016/j.eclinm.2018.07.001.

128. Vindrola-Padros C, Ramsay AIG, Perry C, et al. Implementing major system change in specialist cancer surgery: The role of provider networks. *J Health Serv Res Policy* 2020; 26: 4–11. https://doi.org/10.1177/1355819620926553.

129. Fulop NJ, Ramsay AI, Vindrola-Padros C, et al. Reorganising specialist cancer surgery for the twenty-first century: A mixed methods evaluation (RESPECT-21). *Implement Sci* 2016; 11: 155. https://doi.org/10.1186/s13012-016-0520-5.

130. Turner S, Ramsay AI, Perry C, et al. Lessons for major system change: Centralisation of stroke services in two metropolitan areas of England. *J Health Serv Res Policy* 2016; 21: 156–65. https://doi.org/10.1177/1355819615626189.

131. McKevitt C, Ramsay AIG, Perry C, et al. Patient, carer and public involvement in major system change in acute stroke services: The construction of value. *Health Expect* 2018; 21: 685–92. https://doi.org/10.1111/hex.12668.

132. Fraser A, Baeza JI, Boaz A. 'Holding the line': A qualitative study of the role of evidence in early phase decision-making in the reconfiguration of stroke services in London. *Health Res Policy Syst* 2017; 15: 45. https://doi.org/10.1186/s12961-017-0207-7.

133. Fraser A, Stewart E, Jones L. The importance of sociological approaches to the study of service change in health care. *Sociol Health Illn* 2019; 41: 1215–20. https://doi.org/10.1111/1467-9566.12942.

134. Fulop NJ, Ramsay AI, Vindrola-Padros C, et al. Centralisation of specialist cancer surgery services in two areas of England: The RESPECT-21 mixed-methods evaluation. *Health Soc Care Deliv Res* 2023; 11(2). https://doi.org/10.3310/QFGT2379.

135. Black GB, Wood VJ, Ramsay AIG, et al. Loss associated with subtractive health service change: The case of specialist cancer centralization. *J Health Serv Res Policy* 2022; 27: 301–12. https://doi.org/10.1177/13558196221082585.

136. Smith T, Fowler-Davis S, Nancarrow S, Ariss SMB, Enderby P. Leadership in interprofessional health and social care teams: A literature review. *Leadersh Health Serv* 2018; 31: 452–67. https://doi.org/10.1108/LHS-06-2016-0026.

137. Lyubovnikova J, West MA. Why teamwork matters: Enabling health care team effectiveness for the delivery of high-quality patient care. In: Salas E, Tannenbaum S, Cohen D, Latham G, eds. *Developing and Enhancing Teamwork in Organizations*. San Francisco, CA: Jossey Bass; 2013: 331–72. www.researchgate.net/profile/Michael_West12/pub lication/285218775_Team_working_and_effectiveness_in_health_care/links/593696fda6fdccb0996184d4/Team-working-and-effectiveness-in-health-care.pdf (accessed 22 May 2023).

138. West MA, Lyubovnikova J. Illusions of team working in health care. *J Health Organ Manag* 2013; 27: 134–42. https://doi.org/10.1108/14777261311311843.

139. Lyubovnikova J, West MA, Dawson JF, Carter MR. 24-karat or fool's gold? Consequences of real team and co-acting group membership in healthcare organizations. *Eur J Work Organ Psychol* 2015; 24: 929–50. https://doi.org/10.1080/1359432X.2014.992421.

140. Wranik WD, Price S, Haydt SM, et al. Implications of interprofessional primary care team characteristics for health services and patient health outcomes: A systematic review with narrative synthesis. *Health Policy* 2019; 123: 550–63. https://doi.org/10.1016/j.healthpol.2019.03.015.

141. West M, Almo-Metcalfe B, Dawson J, et al. *Effectiveness of Multi-Professional Team Working (MPTW) in Mental Healthcare*. Southampton: National Institute for Health Research; 2012. https://njl-admin.nihr.ac.uk/document/download/2008984 (accessed 22 May 2023).

142. Austin JM, Demski R, Callender T, et al. From board to bedside: How the application of financial structures to safety and quality can drive account-ability in a large health care system. *Jt Comm J Qual Patient Saf* 2017; 43: 166–75. https://doi.org/10.1016/j.jcjq.2017.01.001.

143. Maben J, Ball J, Edmondson AC. Workplace conditions. In: Dixon-Woods M, Brown K, Marjanovic S, et al., eds. *Elements of Improving Quality and Safety in Healthcare*. Cambridge: Cambridge University Press; 2022. https://doi.org/10.1017/9781009363839.

144. Smith T, Fowler Davis S, et al. Towards a theoretical framework for integrated team leadership (IgTL). *J Interprof Care* 2019; 34: 726–36. https://doi.org/10.1080/13561820.2019.1676209.

145. Warwick-Giles L, Checkland K. Integrated care: Using 'sensemaking' to understand how organisations are working together to transform local

health and social care services. *J Health Organ Manag* 2018; 32: 85–100. https://doi.org/10.1108/JHOM-03-2017-0057.

146. Edmondson AC, Harvey J-F. Cross-boundary teaming for innovation: Integrating research on teams and knowledge in organizations. *Hum Resour Manag Rev* 2018; 28: 347–60. https://doi.org/10.1016/j .hrmr.2017.03.002.

147. Øvretveit J. Improvement leaders: What do they and should they do? A summary of a review of research. *BMJ Qual Saf* 2010; 19: 490–2. https://doi.org/10.1136/qshc.2010.041772.

148. Bate P, Robert G, Fulop N, Øvretveit J, Dixon-Woods M. *Perspectives on Context: A Selection of Essays Considering the Role of Context in Successful Quality Improvement*. London: The Health Foundation; 2014. www .health.org.uk/publications/perspectives-on-context (accessed 22 May 2023).

149. Fulop N, Robert G. *Context for Successful Quality Improvement*. London: The Health Foundation; 2015. www.health.org.uk/publications/context-for-successful-quality-improvement (accessed 22 May 2023).

150. Nicolini D, Waring J, Mengis J. Policy and practice in the use of root cause analysis to investigate clinical adverse events: Mind the gap. *Soc Sci Med* 2011; 73: 217–25. https://doi.org/10.1016/j.socscimed.2011.05.010.

151. Smithson R, Richardson E, Roberts J, et al. *Impact of the Care Quality Commission on Provider Performance: Room for Improvement?* London: The King's Fund; 2018. www.kingsfund.org.uk/publications/impact-cqc-provider-performance (accessed 22 May 2023).

152. Steward K. *Exploring CQC's Well-Led Domain: How Can Boards Ensure a Positive Organisational Culture*. London: The King's Fund; 2014. www .kingsfund.org.uk/sites/default/files/field/field_publication_file/explor ing-cqcs-well-led-domain-kingsfund-nov14.pdf (accessed 22 May 2023).

153. Care Quality Commission. *A New Strategy for the Changing World of Health and Social Care: Our Strategy from 2021*. London: CQC; 2021. www.cqc.org.uk/sites/default/files/Our_strategy_from_2021.pdf (accessed 22 May 2023).

154. Rayner M. The Care Quality Commission: A regulatory evolution. *Judicial Rev* 3 April 2022; 27(2): 126–31. https://doi.org/10.1080 /10854681.2022.2111965.

155. Care Quality Commission. *Single Assessment Framework*. www.cqc.org .uk/about-us/how-we-will-regulate/single-assessment-framework (accessed 22 May 2023).

156. NHS England, NHS Improvement. *NHS System Oversight Framework 2021/ 22*. London: NHS England, NHS Improvement; 2021. www.england.nhs.uk/

wp-content/uploads/2021/06/B0693-nhs-system-oversight-framework-2021-22.pdf (accessed 22 May 2023).

157. Barnett RC, Weidenfeller NK. Shared leadership and team performance. *Adv Dev Hum Resour* 2016; 18: 334–51. https://doi.org/10.1177/1523422316645885.

158. Ansell C, Sørensen E, Torfing J. The COVID-19 pandemic as a game changer for public administration and leadership? The need for robust governance responses to turbulent problems. *Publ Manag Rev* 2021; 23: 949–60. https://doi.org/10.1080/14719037.2020.1820272.

159. Scognamiglio F, Sancino A, Caló F, Jacklin-Jarvis C, Rees J. The public sector and co-creation in turbulent times: A systematic literature review on robust governance in the COVID-19 emergency. *Publ Admin* 2 August 2022. www.ncbi.nlm.nih.gov/pmc/articles/PMC9350016/ (accessed 22 May 2023).

160. Mintz LJ, Stoller JK. A systematic review of physician leadership and emotional intelligence. *J Grad Med Educ* 2014; 6: 21–31. https://doi.org/10.4300/JGME-D-13-00012.1.

161. Marchal B, Westhorp G, Wong G, et al. Realist RCTs of complex interventions: An oxymoron. *Soc Sci Med* 2013; 94: 124–8. https://doi.org/10.1016/j.socscimed.2013.06.025.

162. Moore G, Audrey S, Barker M, et al. Process evaluation of complex interventions. *BMJ* 2015; 350: h1258. https://doi.org/10.1136/bmj.h1258.

163. Greenhalgh T, Papoutsi C. Studying complexity in health services research: Desperately seeking an overdue paradigm shift. *BMC Med* 2018; 16: 95. https://doi.org/10.1186/s12916-018-1089-4.

164. Fletcher A, Jamal F, Moore G, et al. Realist complex intervention science: Applying realist principles across all phases of the Medical Research Council framework for developing and evaluating complex interventions. *Evaluation* 2016; 22: 286–303. https://doi.org/10.1177/1356389016652743.

165. Chambers N, Smith J, Proudlove N, et al. Roles and behaviours of diligent and dynamic healthcare boards. *Health Serv Manage Res* 2020; 33: 96–108. https://doi.org/10.1177/0951484819887507.

Cambridge Elements ☰

Improving Quality and Safety in Healthcare

Editors-in-Chief
Mary Dixon-Woods
THIS Institute (The Healthcare Improvement Studies Institute)

Mary is Director of THIS Institute and is the Health Foundation Professor of Healthcare Improvement Studies in the Department of Public Health and Primary Care at the University of Cambridge. Mary leads a programme of research focused on healthcare improvement, healthcare ethics, and methodological innovation in studying healthcare.

Graham Martin
THIS Institute (The Healthcare Improvement Studies Institute)

Graham is Director of Research at THIS Institute, leading applied research programmes and contributing to the institute's strategy and development. His research interests are in the organisation and delivery of healthcare, and particularly the role of professionals, managers, and patients and the public in efforts at organisational change.

Executive Editor
Katrina Brown
THIS Institute (The Healthcare Improvement Studies Institute)

Katrina is Communications Manager at THIS Institute, providing editorial expertise to maximise the impact of THIS Institute's research findings. She managed the project to produce the series.

Editorial Team
Sonja Marjanovic
RAND Europe

Sonja is Director of RAND Europe's healthcare innovation, industry, and policy research. Her work provides decision-makers with evidence and insights to support innovation and improvement in healthcare systems, and to support the translation of innovation into societal benefits for healthcare services and population health.

Tom Ling
RAND Europe

Tom is Head of Evaluation at RAND Europe and President of the European Evaluation Society, leading evaluations and applied research focused on the key challenges facing health services. His current health portfolio includes evaluations of the innovation landscape, quality improvement, communities of practice, patient flow, and service transformation.

Ellen Perry
THIS Institute (The Healthcare Improvement Studies Institute)

Ellen supported the production of the series during 2020–21.

About the Series
The past decade has seen enormous growth in both activity and research on improvement in healthcare. This series offers a comprehensive and authoritative set of overviews of the different improvement approaches available, exploring the thinking behind them, examining evidence for each approach, and identifying areas of debate.

Cambridge Elements ≡

Improving Quality and Safety in Healthcare

Elements in the Series

Printed in the United States
by Baker & Taylor Publisher Services